How To NOT Live In The Toilet When You Have Stomach Parasites

Peter LeGrove

My Bout With Travellers Diarrhea And How I Managed To Get Well Again

Disclaimer

Although the author and publisher have made every effort to ensure that the information in this book was correct at press time, the author and publisher do not assume and hereby disclaim any liability to any party for any loss, damage, or disruption caused by errors or omissions, whether such errors or omissions result from negligence, accident, or any other cause.

This book is for entertainment purposes only. The views expressed are of the author alone and should not be taken as expert advice. The reader is responsible for his own actions. Neither the author nor the publisher assume any liability or responsibility on behalf of the reader and or purchaser of this material.

You must use common sense when treating yourself from any aliments, The author and publisher assume no liability or responsibility for any accidents or anything that happens to you while reading or following this book. The author is not a licensed Medical Practitioner in any country in the world, he is an author writing about what he did to control internal parasites.

The author and publisher claim no responsibility for results obtained while following this book, as everybody is different and is starting at different levels. You the reader are responsibility for your actions and safety while trying to overcome a parasite infection.

Your Free Book

As a way of saying thank you for buying my book I'm offering you a free book.

This book "How To Add Qualifications To Your CV Using FREE Courses" is about what you can learn over the internet for free. It shows you where to go to get Certificates of Accomplishment that you can add to your CV.

Click here and you will be taken to another page where you can download the free book.

Get Your FREE book here

Who Will Benefit From This Book

This book is for everybody as stomach parasites are not confined to the developing world anymore. It doesn't matter where you live, you can still get and possible already have stomach parasites.

If you have uncontrolled diarrhea that will not go away and your doctors do not know what is wrong with you, then you might have stomach parasites. Stomach parasites are notoriously difficult to detect and the damage some parasites cause to your stomach is not good. Also if you are taking anti-diarrhea medicine especially Imodium and other generic brands of loperamide, which is an opioid, to help get you through the day you need to do something different. This book will help.

If you travel overseas to any country, especially a developing country, you need this book as the possibility of picking up a parasite is quite high, but in these countries they usually know which little beast you have and they also know how to treat the invasion. When you arrive back home to your hometown nobody knows what is wrong with you, so it is better to get treated in the country where you got sick.

There are many causes of uncontrolled persistent diarrhea that you can't shake off so do a few things mentioned in the book and see if it makes a difference.

If you are an ESL teacher, a missionary or just a stranger in a strange land then this book could be for you.

How To Use This Book

Start by reading the book and see if it is for you. Then try a few things and see if it makes a difference. This book is basically about taking control of your health and looking after yourself. When you go to the doctor you are one of many patients, but when you start to take control of your own health you are the only one. And with parasites as their symptoms are the same as many other stomach related disorders you could be treated for other aliments you do not have. You need your doctor so you can get the meds because there are a number of special antibiotics just for parasites. Some kill the beast and some don't and in the process between the parasites and the antibiotics your stomach can get pretty messed up.

After you have read the book, decide what you would like to try out and do it but give it tie to work. With spices and supplements there is no instant success, it takes time. Now everybody is different so what helped me might not help you, so try something else. Also if your body is not used to spices and supplements your body will need to get used to them.

I am not a medical practitioner I am just writing about what I did to rid myself of internal parasites.

Also you might need to change your diet as there are certain foods that internal parasites live off so you will need to stop eating some foods.

Conclusion: It Took Me Years To Work This Out.

If you have terrible diarrhea that will not go away try this and see if it makes your life bearable. Crush and dice 4 large cloves of garlic, preferable organic, and leave it sit for over 20 minutes then eat it raw with 1000 to 1500mgs of Vitamin C every night just before you go to bed, so it sits in your stomach all night. This is to kill the beast.

As with all things start in moderation and work up, like start with one clove of garlic and work your way up. I was eating about half a bulb at one stage. When you eat it at night by the time you go to work you do not smell so bad. DO NOT eat garlic before going to work or you will stink the office out.

Also during the day sprinkle one tablespoon of tumeric on some food and eat it, this is to stop inflammation.

Before you eat lunch or dinner drink a tablespoon of Apple Cider Vinegar, this is to try and get your stomach acid up as you need stomach acid to kill the beast.

There are a lot of other things you can try and I recommend you try them as everybody is different and they could work better for you. Vitamin C and crushed garlic worked for me, I hope it works for you too.

This Is My Story:

I spent a bit of time travelling around China and Vietnam and just before I was due to come home I ended up with a bout of diarrhea. I should have know something was wrong as this was not the usual bout of food poisoning. Food poisoning is usually explosive diarrhea that comes on fast then vanishes. Causes a few problems for a few days then it is back to normal. What I had was dysentery style diarrhea that was very awkward, as I had to walk around with a wad of toilet paper stuffed up my butt to catch the drops. I couldn't fart. Anyway that was all I had, no cramps, no nausea, and no pain. I felt OK, I just needed a toilet in very close proximity. I just didn't eat if I had to go out. I used to drink heaps as I needed too as I was in the tropics in summer and I had dysentery. This went on for over a week and I used to take some pills they gave me in China, but there was no change. If I had felt really terrible I would have gone to the doctor, but I didn't think there was any reason too. Anyway I broke my golden rule which is – always go to the doctor in the country you are sick in, as they would most likely know what is wrong with you. When you get back to your home country the doctors usually have absolutely no clue what is wrong with you. I got amoebic dysentery while in the sahara and I went to the doctor there and they knew exactly what was wrong with me and they gave me the correct medicine. Where as one of my friends got very sick in Russia in Leningrad, then he went home and no one knew what was wrong with him. About 2 years later I caught up with him and I told him to go to a Russian doctor. He did and the doctor knew exactly what was wrong with him and gave him the correct medicine and then he was OK. So get checked before you fly home.

Anyway on the flight home I didn't eat anything. I asked for an aisle seat but I couldn't get one. I had a window seat and that meant crawling over two people to get out. So I was very careful and didn't drink very much either. I made it back without too many problems.

I thought I had worms so I took a worm pill but everything was just flying through my system so fast the pill didn't stay in my system long enough to do any good. Anyway I wanted to try out this Diatomaceous Earth stuff which was supposed to be good at getting rid of stomach worms. I thought I had stomach worms of some description. So when I got home I brought a half kilo of Diatomaceous Earth to try it out. And either I didn't have worms or that stuff didn't work very good. I will admit it did settle my stomach, no tummy rumblings at night but it didn't dent the diarrhea. I was taking a tablespoon mixed in a glass of water first thing in the morning and last thing at night for two weeks. Didn't taste too good but I was hoping it would stop the diarrhea but it didn't. So I started checking out the internet and I could have giardia but I didn't have any severe symptoms just diarrhea bordering on dysentery. And the people who ended up with giardia knew they had something. So I was at a bit of a loose end. I thought I had giardia because it can cause lactose intolerance. And drinking milk again was a problem. I never drink milk in Asia as that HT milk is terrible. I was now back into milk country and my diarrhea was not getting better. So I stopped the milk and to stop giardia you need to eat garlic first thing in the morning and then before you go to bed. So I was eating about four cloves of crushed garlic in the morning and again in the evening. And things started to harden up but that didn't last long, then it was back to what it was before. Maybe I didn't have giardia. I kept chewing on garlic for another couple of weeks then I gave up.

Then somebody said I might have a stomach virus as that can cause severe diarrhea. One thing I've taken in the past for stomach acid problems like GERD was a teaspoon of baking soda in a class of water. Here I let the glass sit for about half an hour or longer before drinking it. But there is one severe problem with baking soda and that is you can use it as a cleanse. So that made the situation a lot worse, I had full blown dysentery while this was going on. Vitamin C is very good at stopping a virus so I brought a jar of powered Vitamin C and used a teaspoon in a glass of water. Now on the label it says Vitamin C in large doses can cause diarrhea and sure enough it did. When that happens everything just flies through your system so it doesn't get absorbed. So you are basically wasting it. Anyway I tried half a teaspoon of Vitamin C with half a teaspoon of baking soda to see if that would slow things down but it didn't, so I stopped that and will probably go back when things harden up.

I read somewhere that activated charcoal somehow cleaned a lot of toxic stuff out of your stomach. It somehow bound all the bad bits and they were flushed out of your system with the charcoal. So I started flushing out my system with the charcoal. I took 6 pills in the morning then I waited over two hours before drinking and eating. And the charcoal slowed the through put down somewhat but not completely. It was about this time that I finally worked out I needed fibre in my diet. So I started to get into psyllium husk for fibre and things started to get a lot better. Now this psyllium husk did make a difference, but you have to be careful with this stuff. It is recommended for constipation but fibre helps diarrhea as well. It binds everything together. And also it can swell up inside you as it absorbs moisture and that is where you have to be careful as it can cause a blockage. That was another thing I looked at as diarrhea can be a symptom of a blockage, but not my case. I was still blowing out food that was not digested properly so the through put was still pretty fast.

So far the only combination that controlled the diarrhea was deactivated charcoal and psyllium husk. Now the name Bentonite Clay also popped up as another cure for persistent diarrhea. After trying out Diatomaceous Earth, I am used to eating dirt so I thought I'd try this out. Now with both

Diatomaceous Earth and Bentonite Clay you need the food grade product, so make sure you get food grade as there is also a non food grade product and you don't want that. This Bentonite Clay is very similar to deactivated charcoal, they both absorb things in your body that shouldn't be there. So I was hoping they would pick up and discard what I had. The charcoal was very good and the reports swore this was a lot better. Also Bentonite Clay is similar to psyllium husk as it swells up inside you and can cause a blockage, so be careful and drink lots of water. Both with Bentonite Clay and charcoal you need to take them on an empty stomach and then not eat anything for about two hours. So I took a teaspoon in a glass of water before bed and just after I got up, then I would drink lots of tea to keep the fluids going.

The whole time I had diarrhea I never had very much control over my bodily functions. If I needed to go I had to go and that was it. Many times I was saved by the wad of toilet paper stuffed up my butt. The biggest mistake I made was starting to drink milk again as that threw me back to square one. With me milk and diarrhea do not mix. Also if you have giardia you could end up lactose intolerant as that little evil parasite can do that. I have never had lactose intolerance before so that is why I thought I had giardia. Another thing I noticed is I was eating more and I was feeling hungry all the time. That could be because I wasn't getting many nutrients from the food as it was flying through my system or something else was causing that, like giardia. I don't know.

Also I was looking at gluten which can cause diarrhea and a whole bunch of other problems if you are really sensitive to gluten. We have gluten problems in our family, my brother has it quite bad, my sister eats gluten free stuff and so far if I overdose on gluten I just fall asleep. So I am thinking of giving up eating bread again. I have given up eating bread before but it is quite difficult. Then again if nothing is going to cure me then I'll give up eating bread again and see what happens.

The other thing I'm looking at is fasting. I used to fast very regularly before but I changed my job and now I don't fast as much. Fasting seems to be the cure all for any number of diseases, and if nothing else cures my diarrhea then I'll give fasting another go. Right now I seem to be eating a lot more, I don't know if that is a by-product of the diarrhea or something else. It could be because the food I eat doesn't stay inside me long enough to digest properly therefore I don't get enough nutrients from the food. And as I don't get enough nutrients my body is crying out for more food so it can get more nutrients, a vicious cycle. Also as the Bentonite Clay sucks a lot of particles, whether good or bad, from you colon it is difficult to take vitamin supplements as the Clay will bind to them and excrete them from your system. What I do is drink a glass of Bentonite Clay morning and evening and have my vitamins and any other pills for lunch. Also I usually don't eat breakfast, I try to go as long as I can before eating anything. That still leaves me a window from 12 to 4 pm to take any medicine. But I have found as I drink a lot of tea, both green and black tea with no milk or sugar, in the morning that that can make the diarrhea worse. Like I have dysentary most morning. I don't know if that is due to just drinking too much fluid and no food or it is the diarrhea being diarrhea. Now all I am taking is Bentonite Clay and psyllium husk. I like to take a glass of two teaspoons of psyllium husk in water a couple of hours after the Clay. Also the psyllium husk takes away the feelings of wanting to eat so it stops you feeling hungry. This article here got me more into psyllium husk and it turns out this stuff is very healthy. I made the mistake of not buying organic and the one I got has sugar in it, which is not the healthiest thing you can eat. So next time I'll just buy organic psyllium husk by itself. Some brands come out with artificial sugar and that is not always the healthiest option either. I have a severe sweet tooth so I try to keep away from sugar.

With diarrhea it is actually quite difficult to find out what is working and what is not, because you do not know how long it takes for the food you eat to pass through your system. So if you change anything, like what you eat you do not know if it works or if it is something else. To find out how long it takes food to pass through you I use deactivated charcoal because you can see when it comes out. I used to eat six capsules first thing in the morning as you shouldn't eat or drink anything for two hours before and two hours after digesting the charcoal. And then wait till it comes out. It usually took 11 hours to pass through my system. That gives you an idea of how long to wait to see if your new treatment is working or not. I used to do everything for a week, like one week of taking Diatomaceous Earth twice daily morning and evening to see if works or not. Then one week of psyllium husk and then one week of the two combined to see if the combination works better. You have to do your own trial and error on this one. But if you are fairly sure what you are doing doesn't make any difference or makes it worse try something new.

Another thing that is very good for diarrhea is probotics. The problem with probiotics is they usually come from milk and if you are sensitive to lactose, milk probiotics could be a problem. So I stuck to fermented vegetables. Fermented vegetables usually take a month to make and the longer you leave them the more probiotic they get. You can buy them from the health food shop as well as the supermarket. One of the best is kim chi, the fermented vegetables from Korea, so head down to your local Korean supermarket and pick some up. If you are going to make your own expect a month before you can start eating them. They are easy to make. I usually make sauerkraut from cabbage, easy to make and it tastes good. If you have an upset stomach you do need probiotics. If you can stomach milk based probiotics then go for it. Just eating non sweetened yoghurt should make a difference. The acidophilus and lactobacillus organisms in the yoghurt are what you want, and good quality unsweetened yoghurt should have them.

One of the worst things to come out of this diarrhea is lack of control. All the other times I've been able to hold it in but this time I have very little control. If I feel like I got to go I got to go, there is no waiting around. So I walk around with a wad of toilet paper stuffed up my butt to catch the drops. That is a must. Things are not good. Another thing that really upsets me is when it looks good and things are starting to harden up. Then the next time it is back to water and slops. Usually the first time in the morning its good but the next time it is not. Maybe not moving settles it all down and then after I get up and with the movement it goes back to water. Very sad.

Now I have started on the garlic again. Same as last time I take 5 to 6 cloves crushed for 15 minutes just after I get up and again just before I go to bed. I did make one very serious mistake I brought some yoghurt and now I am back to lactose intolerant and everything has gone back to water. I now have to wait until the yoghurt is out of my system so I can find out if the garlic is working or not. I did read on the internet that grapefruit is good for internal parasites but I am nearly out of grapefruit, so I don't know what to do there.

After yesterday's bout of complete water for poo, this morning I had the first near normal poo I've had in three months. So it is time to start looking at what I eat. No one anywhere on the internet ever mentioned doing a food log so now I am going to start one just to see if what I eat is making a difference. Yesterday for the first time I had grapefruit for breakfast, ate seeds and all everything except the skin. Maybe that made a difference. Anyway I started the day with my crushed garlic. I crush the garlic cut it into little pieces wait 15 minutes then eat it. If some gets stuck in my throat I drink a little water. When I eat the garlic I just swallow it, I don't try to chew it or anything just swallow it. This way you do not get the big garlic breath. Sometimes I've noticed little chopped up bits of garlic floating in the toilet bowl, so sometimes it goes straight through without even being digested. Not good. Then I eat nothing and drink nothing for 2 hours. That is every morning with garlic. When I was drinking my bentonite clay mixture I always used to drink plenty of black or green tea. With the charcoal I always waited 2 to 3 hours before eating or drinking to give it a head start and time to clean out my stomach.

Now back to yesterday. After the 2 hour wait for the garlic to get a head start I drank about 3 to 5 cups of tea. Then about 4 hours after getting up I had a grapefruit, ate everything except the skin. That was breakfast. For lunch I had steak on toast with a bowl of sauerkraut. And one toast and marmalade and one toast and raspberry jam. Around 5 oclock I had 2 teaspoons of psyllium husk mixed with a cup of yoghurt, my last little cup of yoghurt. I am not getting any more yoghurt or milk until my stomach is way back to normal. For dinner around 7 oclock I ate sardines on 2 pieces of toast with tomato and again one toast and marmalade and one toast and raspberry jam. I am trying to finish up the bread so I can live without bread to see if that makes a difference. If I stop the toast that should lower my sugar levels. Through the day I eat a few slices of cheese and a few dates and drink lots of tea.

In the morning my poo was nearly normal and I could control it but as the day worn on it started to deteriorate back to nearly water and I couldn't hold it back. That is usually what happens during the day.

Well today started off really good with one good poo to start the day. It was a bit bloaty and a bit farty but it was reasonable solid. What I ate yesterday was very similar to the day before. I started the day with crushed garlic, then waited 2 hours before having something to drink. I had about 4 cups of tea then a grapefruit for breakfast. This time for lunch I had 2 teaspoons of psyllium husk mixed with coconut cream, not a bad mixture and some cashew nuts and almonds. Now around 3 oclock I cooked up half an ox kidney with onion fried on toast, not bad at all, and finished it off with one toast and marmalade and one toast and raspberry jam. Around 5 another 2 teaspoons of psyllium husk mixed with coconut cream. Now I have run out of coconut cream. For dinner around 7 I boiled up a mixture of kale and silverbeet and again had sardines on toast with sliced tomato and another slice of toast and marmalade. Hopefully today I will run out of bread. It could be quite difficult to live without bread.

As most of the winter kale and cabbages are going to seed I think I'll bring out the juicer and see how much juice I can get out of what is left. Today is Sunday so no garlic as I go to church, so I started the day off with a cup of tea. Just before I left to go to church I had some psylliun husk with coconut cream. Really the whole morning was not very good as I had to run out of church to go to the toilet. So maybe the psyllium husk or no garlic or whatever didn't work very well. Anyway being a Sunday things were slightly different. I started off with a grapefruit then I finished off the last of the bread. Had a piece of steak for lunch and vegetables for dinner and no garlic before bed. My body was pretty messed up so maybe garlic was the way to go. The next day I started off with garlic and we got off to a good start. No bread now so I'll see if that makes a difference. Breakfast was back to raisin bran with a couple of scoops of husk with coconut cream and no sweetened yoghurt. Three sausages for lunch and some boiled then fried potatoes with broccoli for dinner.

I was reading on the net and the article said giardia lives off sugar. That is the second time I've had a connection between sugar and giardia. I figured I should lay off the sugar but I have a severe sweet tooth. And I just realized the brand of psyllium husk I have has over 50% sugar so that is not going to help. I have to knock off the carbs. Bread has gone but I still have lots of lollies and chocolate left. So I will have to do something about that. I brought some low fat unsweetened yoghurt with added probiotics so I'll see if that makes a difference. For dessert I had a cup of yoghurt, coconut cream and two teaspoons of psyllium husk, and 4 cloves of garlic before going to bed. I'll look into that sugar connection because sugar is something a number of diseases and bugs live off, cancer for example and now giardia.

Well this morning was the best morning I've had for a very long time, maybe giving up the bread helped or was it the probiotic yoghurt or the garlic started kicking in I don't know. Anyway something happened and I hope it keeps happening.

I didn't have any garlic last night and today I am paying for it. Generally speaking I am a lot better whether that is due to no bread or probiotic yoghurt or something else I don't know. Also last night I went on a sweet binge and that is not good. I have to do something about the amount of sugar I am eating my psyllium husk has over half sugar, I should have realised when I brought a popular brand name, I was advised to buy organic. I should have as it would have been a lot cheaper per unit of psyllium husk. Here I paid more for sugar than psyllium husk. Anyway I think I have finally got it under control, yesterday was a good. And so far today is a good day I had some garlic this morning and none last night. Last night I had some yoghurt and husk just before going to bed and that settled everything. But those were the last of the good days. Now it is back to what it was like before, which is basically very little control over my bodily functions. For the whole time I've had this bout of diarrhea I have only overflowed the wad of toilet paper stuffed up my butt three times. Which is pretty darn good considering I can't fart and I have intermittent bloating. So now I have to reconsider what I have eating. Maybe I ate too much yoghurt and that clicked in the lactose intolerance.

The recommendation is only half a cup of yoghurt each time, but as is usually the case when something starts to work you overdo it and then you are back to square one and that is where I am now. I might have to lay off the fried food. The recommendation is for a low fat diet and I live off lard. Now I might have to go back to frying food in coconut oil and olive oil and or butter. I still live off streak and sausages with vegetables and home made sauerkraut. I brought some organic psyllium husk and as soon as I have finished the sugar one I'll start the organic and see if that makes a difference. I am very disappointed in the brand name psyllium husk because of the sugar content. And at the supermarket I see the price has gone down possible because they are not selling it and I am not going to buy it again. Anyway things are still not good so I don't know what has happened. As giardia seems to live off sugar it is time to knock sugar on the head. I started the new organic psyllium husk with probiotic yoghurt but it didn't seem to do any good. Also now I am eating more than I usually do so that might not help. If I can't kill the beast by stopping sugar then I'll get into fasting. I've already given up bread which is carbohydrate and turns to sugar in your body, so now I just have to lay off the raisin bran and the sugar husk and hopefully that will help. At the moment the only thing that makes a difference is raw crushed garlic so I have started that again as well as bentonite clay. I might have to drop the morning coffee as it is acidic and the beast likes an acid environment. I might try a half teaspoon of baking soda and Vitamin C and see if that will lower acidity and increase alkalinity in my stomach. The beast doesn't like probiotics, alkaline, garlic but it loves sugar, so I have to rearrange my eating habits to oppose the beast. Also I've noticed the garlic I eat does not get digested, it just floats around the toilet bowl the same as I ate it, chopped up into little bits. It must just flow straight through my system, I wonder if it does any good. Now I have changed and I mix psyllium husk with chia seeds and probiotic yoghurt. And at the moment that seems to be the best but for how long.

So far not much has changed I've added Cayenne pepper and apple cider vinegar to the mix. I've had stomach acid problems for years now and I have usually used plain old baking soda to keep my heart burn and reflux under control. I've known for a while that stomach acid problems can be caused by too little acid. Now with some vegetables passing through me with what looks like not being digested I thought I would add more acid to the mix to see if it makes a difference. And that is the opposite of what I should be doing as the beast likes an acid environment. But I think that is to do with an acid environment caused by eating too much acidic foods and not stomach acid. Anyway I broke down and bread on special enticed me so I brought two loaves, big mistake my stomach has not been the same since. When I have finished eating those two loaves I'll not buy any more. I think there might be a glutin thing in my system somewhere. If the beast can turn you into lactose intolerant then it might be able to do something with gluten. And I went from unsweetened probiotic yoghurt to the usual yoghurt and my lactose intolerance really kicked in so things are going backwards at the moment. Also I'm getting slightly run down and depression is creeping in as I have been thinking of going to the doctor. But I don't know if that will make a difference. That or go on a five day fast which would be the most healthy option. I added the Cayenne pepper as that is a general health option used in a number of tropical countries for bug control, so I'll see if that helps. Actually thinking back I should have added the new stuff separately then I could judge if they made a difference. Right now if I start to improve I will not know which one made the difference. I've also added cinnamon to my morning mixture of yoghurt, phyllism husk, chia seeds and cayenne pepper. I found a couple of little packets of cinnamon while I was looking for the cayenne pepper so I thought I'll use them.

Well things haven't been too good lately. I went on a sugar binge for a couple of days and the beast loved it. Now I don't know if I went on the binge because I was depressed or my sugar cravings got the better of me. Depression set in for about a week as the insidious beast was winning and everything I did had no effect. I think what happens is, the beast comes in waves where it must overproduce little beasts and they take control in your stomach until your immune system kicks in and kicks them out. But it doesn't kick them all out and the ones that are left come back with a vengeance and create havoc for a while. And that is when depression sets in. One of the reasons depression set in is because I had a few new symptoms, I started feeling nauseous and I had pain in my leg. I felt like I was going to puke but didn't. Anyway that went away after a few days and the pain in my knee vanished as suddenly as it had started, but the excessive diarrhea persisted. I don't know why the pain in my leg happened. I hurt my planter fascitis in my foot a while back sprinting across the football field. Your planter fascitis is the tendon that runs from the back of your heel under your foot to your toes, and you don't want to damage it as it hurts like hell and it is very difficult to get comfortable with this aliment. Mainly because you are on your feet most of the time and when you drive it can make it worse. And that is something you also don't want because when it is resting it hurts the most. In the mornings after sleeping you can hardly put your foot on the floor it hurts so much. You have to stretch it and walk on it to make it feel better. And hopefully after a couple of months it will be back to normal. Now because my immune system is constantly under attack and I probably have excess inflammation in my body my planter fascitis is taking longer to heal. My foot has been hurting for months now so I am used to that, but this time my knee started hurting, and that is a new one. Even if I just rested my arm on my knee it would start to hurt. I was starting to wonder what it was, I thought it might be arthritis or something like that then it vanished. Also it might have been because I am limping a little I might have put more strain on my knee and that caused the problem, but we will never know as it went away. Now because of my planter fascitis I can't run or do too many exercises so I don't know if that is a bad thing or not.

Doing exercises does increase inflammation in your body but there are still many benefits to a good exercise program. And I used to run and do exercises most mornings until the beast got the better of me. I'll go back to exercising as soon as I can as I miss it but I don't want to overdo it as that could put more strain on my overtaxed body, and the beast is causing my immune system and my inflammation system to work overtime.

And then I somehow managed to stop eating the good food, no more garlic and bentonite clay and hello more bread and sugar foods like jam and marmalade and packets of sweets. One new thing I am doing is eating organic coconut oil, a large teaspoon first thing in the morning. I also mix a teaspoon of butter and a teaspoon of coconut oil and about a third of a teaspoon of cayenne pepper in my morning coffee. I don't know if it does any good but it tastes good. I think the cayenne pepper is making a difference and sometimes I sprinkle too much on my food and I have trouble eating it. She is pretty hot stuff.

Well something must be going right I feel the best I have felt since this started, except for some muscle pains and flash headaches, I feel really good. All I am doing now is half a dozen cloves of garlic at night before I go to bed, and in the morning a very large teaspoon of coconut oil. Then I don't eat or drink anything for over four hours. When I do eat I just smother the food in cayenne pepper so it is a little too hot to eat then I eat it. And I feel terrific, I still have diarrhea but it is controllable. And I broke down and brought a parasite cleanse from the local health shop. This has the same ingredients as Hulda Clark's Parasite cleanse so I'll see if it makes a difference.

Also this phase could be the beast's downtime where the lot that has been terrorizing me die off and now we just wait for the new bunch to take hold and start terrorizing me. So if I start using the parasite cleanse now it might actually help. Well yesterday might have been the best day so far but that is the end of it, today I was back to near water and it was water at times. I am lucky I still have a wad of toilet paper stuffed up my butt or I would have had a few near misses today. I don't know if it is the new parasite mixture I just brought or something else. I'll have to wait and see on that one. Or it could be the beast is back with a vengeance and making up for lost time. I could be my own worst enemy here, I'm back on the bread and I've stocked up on chocolate as it was on special as well as biscuits. I haven't started on the biscuits yet but I am chewing away on the chocolate, plus I am using that sugar psyllium husk that I am not too happy about but I'll finish using it up and not buy it again. And I have run out of the sugarless probiotic yoghurt and I am onto ordinary yoghurt which is nowhere near as healthy as the probiotic stuff. That could be one reason why my diarrhea has returned as I am still lactose intolerant. The probiotic yoghurt didn't affect me so much. So I have to rethink what I eat. The bread has to go but that is easier said than done.

Things seem to be getting better, I'm still eating four or five crushed gloves of garlic at night and a big teaspoon of coconut oil in the morning. I add Cayenne pepper to most meals, I even put some in the yoghurt, psyllium husk, cinnamon, nutmeg and raw milk mixture that at the moment doesn't affect my lactose intolerance. I've also added sauerkraut to most hot food at dinner time now. And with all this I am the best I have felt for a long time, even the diarrhea is controllable. I still don't know if I have killed the beast but I might have him on the run.

I still haven't started doing my exercises yet but I am working up to it. My foot is still sore but I need to get back into exercising again. At the moment I am loading up every meal and also in coffee with Cayenne pepper. I was feeling so good that I stopped eating garlic at night then I stopped coconut oil in the mornings. In the morning everything was good but in the afternoon all hell broke loose and I nearly lived in the toilet and that continued on to the next day. But I still feel good and my tummy has stopped rumbling. So maybe it is just lactose intolerance kicking in as I have been eating a lot of junk food lately and the dip was made from cream. To be honest I have probably eaten more junk food this last week that I have for a very long time. I might be able to get hold of some raw goats milk if I can find the place, then I can find out if it is lactose intolerance or the beast is back. Also my immune system might have got on top of it, about time I've had it for nearly six months. I'll have to start eating garlic again at night because it settles my stomach in the morning.

Now I'm just running in and out of the toilet all morning. Maybe the beast is back. Now I'm trying to chew my food longer to try and digest it more as I am most likely suffering from malabsorption. I just don't have the energy I used to have. And sometimes some food is just not digested at all. I don't eat the garlic I just swallow it. And there were times when the garlic just went straight through. It looked like it had never been touched. Another food that went straight through was chard or silverbeet depending on which country you are in. It looks like it is the vegetables that are not digested. It can be difficult to try and find out what food is causing the problems because it can be difficult to work out when you ate what. I like to know how long food takes to go through me and right now it is pretty fast. And to top it off I don't feel sick I have no hurt stomach or any pain, except for my foot which is still a hotbed for inflammation. I have started doing exercises again but not everyday, I have to give time for my body to recover as I haven't doing them for a while. I must have a lot of inflammation in my body as my planter fascitis is causing my foot to swell up. Inflammation usually means you immune system is working overtime to keep your body healthy. Since my immune system is battling the giardia that is causing inflammation in my foot. And my foot has been swollen for about a month now. So I have to build up my immune system and that could mean more zinc and more vitamin C.

Yesterday was a good day, I only went to the toilet 5 times, 3 in the morning and 2 in the afternoon and only one time in the afternoon would be considered serious diarrhea, the others were reasonable and controllable. At the moment I am not taking anything to control the beast. I eat 2 or 3 grapefruit for breakfast and that is it. I will start eating garlic again in the evening so far that is one of the few things that has been good to me. Now I can actually have a pee standing usually I had to sit down as I would be pooing myself at the same time. So things are looking up. If I could lay off the sugar and the bread I might get somewhere. I did read somewhere that one women who had giardia and was pregnant didn't want to take Flagil because of the baby, just stopped sugar and lived of kale juice. And that got rid of the beast. Most of my kale has gone to seed now but there is a little bit left. So I should try that.

Today wasn't too good so I took a hand full of Activated Charcoal and it took 10 hours to go through me. I still have problems with diarrhea but it is usually to do with too much air in the system. When I go to the toilet my poo is interspaced with air, so I have to stop the bloating somehow. If I didn't have the air things would be a lot better. Today I went to the toilet four times two in the morning and two in the afternoon. The worst thing is after I go to the toilet I never feel empty, I always feel like there is more to come. And there is. Before I'd go once a day and that was it. I cleaned myself completely out, but now I sometimes have to go four times before I feel empty, and it is always the same, too much air. The problem is the bloating, if I didn't have the bloating I would think it would be a lot better. I just have to get rid of the air as well as the poo. I've actually given up for a bit now, no garlic, no coconut oil, no Bentonite Clay only Cayenne pepper and then when I have finished all the yoghurt, all the bread and the sweets I should be able to start again. There is no point really in trying to stop the beast when I am feeding it sugars and milk.

Yesterday was a terrible day, I went to the toilet so many times I lost count could have been over ten. I don't know what went wrong or what I had eaten but it was not good. I didn't drink any milk so it wasn't lactose. So I had 5 cloves of crushed and diced garlic before I went to bed. I have to bring my body back under some control. I might be all the chocolate and sweets I am eating.

Things seemed to have calmed down a bit, I'm starting to take stock on what I am eating. I have started drinking a glass of Bentonite Clay in the mornings as well as crushed garlic at night and I'm feeling a hell of a lot better. And I am not living in the toilet. I'm starting to feel a lot better now, it could be I'm getting better or it is just a cycle in the lifestyle of the beast. Now I am using Tumeric in my coffee along with butter, coconut oil and a pinch of Cayenne Pepper. I will now put Tumeric on my food like I do with Cayenne Pepper and see if that helps. I think I should build up my immune system to combat the beast. Also it is difficult to know what works and what doesn't as sometimes it could just be the lifestyle of the beast.

There are times when I feel really good and others when I am just crap and I think that might be the beast not what I am doing. Now I am starting to get heartburn from eating garlic late at night. Last two nights I've had it and that is a new symptom. Also I've been feeling really good, but I still start the day off with my tummy still rumbling away. That has been going on as long as I have had this. When I was taking Diatomaceous Earth that actually stopped the rumblings. I might try Bentonite Clay at night and see if that makes a difference. Alternate between Clay and garlic. If the heartburn turns into a regular thing I might have to drop the garlic. I can only eat garlic at night as I stink the place out during the day. Now the schedule is garlic at night and some mornings a tablespoon of coconut oil and other mornings a tablespoon of

Bentonite Clay in a glass of water. And whether I am controlling the beast or it is just a lull in its lifestyle, I don't know but I am feeling really good. Now I have under 5 poos a day which is a hell of a lot better than living in the toilet.

Got off to a bad start today, I felt really good in the morning, no tummy rumblings. I ate a tablespoon of coconut oil. But the beast must have come back as I had controllable diarrhea. I had to go to the toilet three times in three hours. Then two more times before lunch Not good. But it wasn't bad diarrhea, it was controllable and didn't cause any problems. Yesterday I brought a packet of sweet lollies that might have something to do with it. Also I am adding up to three teaspoons of tumeric a day to my food and that might have an effect on me as my body is not used to it. Also I am eating a lot of tinned beetroot as it was on special and I am waiting for my beetroot kvass to ferment. I am waiting for my other batch of sauerkraut to ferment too so I am not eating too many probiotics at the moment. I had a bowl of natural yoghurt with psyllium husk and I might be reacting to the lactose. Getting healthy is a bitch.

Well I somehow think I might have got on top of the beast, I only went to the toilet three times yesterday and that is a record. And I can actually fart which is something that was not safe to do last week. The main changes are: I am eating more raw vegetables, less bread and milk products and less sweets. I try to eat four to five big cloves of garlic every night. The only time I don't is when it is too late to eat it. I try to eat the garlic about an hour before I go to bed. But my poo is still the same which is still all different, from floating to semi runny and everything in between. So now I am waiting for that to change back to what is was before I say I am back to normal.

In the mornings my stomach is rumbling pretty noisily but it is controllable diarrhea, other than the noise that is all, I don't feel any serious urges to run to the toilet so I don't know what is going on.

At the moment I am eating crushed garlic at night and drinking a tablespoon of Bentonite Clay soaked overnight in water in the morning. I might drink the Bentonite Clay at night and see if that makes a difference. I've still got weird and wonderful poo and as soon as that gets back to normal I'd say the beast is gone but at the moment I don't think so. Well I don't think the beast has gone, last night I drank a tablespoon of Bentonite Clay before bed and woke up with diarrhea so I had another tablespoon as soon as I got up so I'll have to see what happens.

I've been ODing on sugar for the last couple of days that might have something to do with the resurgence of the beast. I have a problem with a sweet tooth and that has to go. I've stopped buying bread but that hasn't stopped me eating it, but it has slowed me down somewhat. Actually it happens when other people buy me lunch, they are so used to eating bread they think everybody still eats it. I've nearly laid off the yoghurt but now I already have diarrhea I may as well have some more yoghurt. Yesterday was a really bad day, I had diarrhea all day so I ate 4 cloves of garlic and this morning a tablespoon of coconut oil and so far things are better today. So maybe I'll stay with garlic and coconut oil, that combination works the best. I'm also eating more raw vegetables like kale leaves, pumpkin leaves and strawberry leaves and that might also help. I've given up the sweets but I've started eating biscuits again, not good as they contain both gluten and sugar.

The very worst thing is in the morning I have to go to the toilet to poo four times.

Before I only went once a day but now because of the beast or whatever I have to go three or four times before I am cleaned out. Usually it is a mixture of air and poo and it is half runny, not quite diarrhea but working on it. Also some food is not digested like before. I try to try to chew my food longer but I have to think consciously about chewing more. I think that might have something to do with the undigested food as well as the beast. I do drink apple cider vinegar mixed with tea to add to my stomach acid but I don't know if that is working.

Well I think the beast is back but not with a vengeance, today for some reason I lived part time in the toilet but it was more to do with bloating than diarrhea. I couldn't really trust myself to fart so I had to go to the toilet each time I got bloated and blow out some air and a bit of water. More annoying than anything else. Now I still eat garlic at night but now in the morning I have a teaspoon of Manuka Honey +10 that is supposed to be as good as an antibiotic. The same as with the coconut oil, nothing to eat or drink for four hours I've had Flagil before but back in the day I think there was more active ingredient in the pills as it was classed as a carcinogenic, that means it can cause cancer and also you couldn't drink alcohol when you were on the pills because it would make you sicker. Now I think it is a class 2 antibiotic which means it is safe for pregnant women so it is definitely not as unhealthy as it was before, and that is probably why giardia is very possibly antibiotic resistant, as it doesn't work on everybody. Anyway I've had this bout of giardia for nearly six months so either my immune system is not up to par or I could have an antoimmune problem linked to gluten as my brother is gluten intolerant, something like leaky gut or irritable bowel syndrome or something like that. I just don't feel sick, I'm doing my exercises most days but my foot still hurts which could mean I have too much inflammation in my body. If my foot healed up I could start running again. I'll keep taking the Manuka Honey for a week and see if it makes any difference. Maybe the sugar in the honey is just feeding the beast. Now I try to limit my gluten intake like I have nearly stopped bread, now I am working on other gluten products. Also I mix a half a teaspoon of Cayenne pepper and two teaspoons of tumuric with every meal and I think that is what is holding me together.

Now I don't know what has happened but my tummy keeps rumbling and the noise actually woke me up one night, but I didn't have to rush off to the toilet so it was just the noise. Anyway I was back to water diarrhea that was controllable and I don't know why, maybe the beast is back.

I kept taking a teaspoon of Manuka Honey in the morning and then I'd wouldn't eat or drink anything till lunchtime, and I thought I'd found a new cure for the beast. Everything was going extremely well until one morning I woke up and my tummy was doing some serious rumblings and I mean serious constant noise and it was a made rush for the toilet and this time I was back to water and this time it was not very controllable. This continued all day until I went to bed. And the next day I was fine. Now the only change in my diet was I binged out on biscuits and I was eating a lot of sweet corn as it is in season. So I don't know if the beast is back or the biscuits were off, but I had a terrible day. With this Manuka Honey I thought it was similar to the red grape cancer treatment I read about somewhere on the internet. Cancer loves sugar so it eats the red grapes and in doing so it also eats the cancer medicine that effectively kills of the cancer. And I was thinking that is the same as with Manuka

Honey. The beast loves sugar so it eats the honey and in doing so it ingests the antibiotic in the honey that hopefully kills it, but it was not meant to be. Anyway I have a few more teaspoons left in the jar so I think I'll alternate between honey, coconut oil and Bentonite Clay and see if that helps. Also I am regularly doing my exercises but I still can't start running as my foot is still swollen up a little bit and it still hurts.

Well things went from good to bad nearly overnight, the next day was good but after that all hell broke loose. It was the worst bout I had had so far. I had nausea and aches and pains. I couldn't even do my exercises. My stomach was rumbling constantly and I used to wake up to the sound of my tummy rumbling and carrying on. Things were so bad I was day dreaming about going to the doctor and asking for some Flagil. I was ill and this lasted for about 4 days. I lived in the toilet and didn't go anywhere without a wad of toilet paper stuffed up my butt, it was just not safe. I didn't drink any milk or dairy but I did eat some corn and that might have thrown me off kilter as corn turns to sugar after you eat it. Anyway it was so bad I started re reading up my webpages about giardia and I found some new things that I could do. Like mixing Cayenne pepper with the manuka +10 honey and eating it together, also mixing Cayenne pepper with coconut oil to make it a bit more potent. And mixing psyllium husk with Bentonite clay and drinking or eating it together. Now I am trying these out and so far everything is good, but this might just be a lull in the life cycle of the beast.

I still don't know if I've killed the beast but I do feel a hell of a lot better. I did have my first solid poo for about six months, so things might be happening but it has since gone back to semi solid. Also I had one day where I could fart without fear, now that was a first for a long time. At the moment I'm eating cayenne pepper with manuka honey first thing in the morning, then two to three hours later I mix cayenne pepper with coconut oil and eat that. I don't eat or drink anything for as long as I can and sometimes I can last up to six hours before having a cup of tea or coffee. On the third morning I'll have a tablespoon of Bentonite Clay mixed with psyllium husk and after two hours I'll start drinking tea. This day is the day I catch up on all the liquid I have not been drinking. I am still eating three to four cloves of crushed and diced garlic every night. Also another reason I think I might have conquered the beast is I don't sleep as much as I have for the last six months. When the beast was causing my immune system to work overtime I needed rest but now I don't seem to need sleep so much. I still binge out on biscuits but not so much and I do eat sour dough bread which is supposed to be the best bread for gluten sensitivity. I have somehow managed to get off the sweets and lollies so that is a plus. I've also started doing my exercises quite regularly but not as often or as hard as before.

So far things are looking good but I don't think I've killed the beast, too much is still the same even though I don't have severe diarrhea. I might have to lay off the cayenne pepper as too much hot stuff can cause diarrhea just to cool down your butt. So instead of eating both honey and coconut oil each day I'll only eat one a day. One day honey and the next day coconut, both mixed with cayenne pepper and the day after that Bentonite Clay with psyllium husk. And see if that makes a difference. Also I'm thinking of bringing in frozen cod liver capsules. The theory behind this is when the capsules are frozen they get further down your digestive tract before the oil is released. And they are supposed to coat the beast with oil making it easier to eliminate the cysts from your body.

Sounds good and I like cod liver oil. So I'll give it a go.

Anyway I started on the frozen cod liver oil capsules and I ended up with a massive dose of diarrhea the next day. I don't know if they are related. Tonight I'll eat garlic and tomorrow I'll take another eight or so frozen capsules and see what happens.

I have come to the conclusion the beast is back but not as bad as before. Most things are controllable. I had one night of constant tummy rumbling and carrying on. It was the worst the rumblings have ever got. If I was laying on my back or right side they were worse that if I was laying on my front or left side, so I managed to get some sleep. No running off to the toilet or anything like that, but I have had controllable diarrhea since then. Anyway I have started frozen fish oil capsules so I'll have to wait and see if they make a difference. When I was in one of my severe depression stages I went out and brought some Oreganio Oil as that is supposed to help kill the best but I haven't started using it yet. I think I might mix a couple of drops in morning honey and coconut mix to see what happens. I only need a couple of drops as it is so strong. Anyway that is in the next couple of days.

I've had quite bad diarrhea for about a week now and it is more annoying than anything else as I have to keep running to the toilet just to fart. Anyway my sweet tooth has taken over so that could be the reason I've had a good bout of diarrhea. It is quite strange really as everything I did to stop the beast did nothing. I ate garlic every night and in the mornings I would either eat honey and cayenne pepper or coconut oil and cayenne pepper and nothing stopped the diarrhea. I started taking eight frozen cod liver oil capsules in the morning and that didn't stop the diarrhea. I have been on a sugar binge for nearly a week but this time I ate some sweets everyday. Usually I just pig out for one day then I run out of sweets, but this time I parked myself in front of the TV and just ate sweets most nights. So I was either just feeding the beast or the beast is back with a vengence. Now I have stopped the sweets as I have run out and we'll see what happens. I didn't eat any bread or milk products the whole week so hopefully it is the sugar and now I hope I can get back to normal. I had serious tummy rumblings the whole week, it was quite embarrassing at times.

So now I'm trying out this Oil of Oregano and see if that makes a difference. A lot of people have said it does work as long as you get the undiluted stuff. Now this stuff is strong so be careful, you have been warned. They recommend 4 to 6 drops but start with 1 or 2 as it is a very acquired taste and to make sure it will not cause any problems start with one drop. I mixed it with coconut oil to thin it down and it was still strong. Anyway the downside to this is, like an antibiotic, it can kill off your gut microflora so you need to stock up on probiotics and fermented foods to replace what the Oil of Oregano kills off. And you need an excellent stomach to get on top of the beast and that usually means probiotics and or fermented vegetables.

My tummy still rumbles something terrible at night so I am not sure what is going on, but the oil of oregano might be clicking in. I have stopped nearly everything, no garlic, no coconut, no honey only tumeric, cayenne pepper and bentonite clay. I am also taking about half a dozen frozen cod liver oil capsules about an hour before I go to bed. I do not know if that is making a difference. So we'll see what happens now. I must admit the first couple of times I used oil of oregano I could feel my kidneys like something was going on there but it was not serious I hope and they calmed down. I checked the internet and oil of oregano can cause kidney stones to come out. So hopefully that wasn't it as the last thing I want now is kidney stones. My immune system is not exactly in top form at the moment so I don't want to cause any problems there. Right now I put two drops of oil of oregano in a drink of orange with a little apple cider vinegar. Tastes terrible but I hope it does some good. At the moment it is not I had a terrible night last night had to run off to the toilet three times. That might have something to do with the two Hot Cross Buns I had after dinner. I have problems with gluten and that was the first bread I'd eaten for a long time. So I can't blame the beast for that I don't think, but I did feel nauseous so the beast might had something to do with that. For breakfast I had a glass of Bentonite Clay and Psyllium Husk hoping that will clean out the system, but we'll have to wait and see on that one. Now I was reading on a facebook group about giardia and one of the guys said he cured his giardia using wheat germ. Now I have never heard of that so I went and brought some to try it out. Because my tummy was rumbling something terrible in the mornings I went back on the 4 cloves of crushed garlic at night and that seemed to have calmed it down a lot. So now some mornings when I have Bentonite Clay and Psyllium Husk I mix in the Wheat Germ and I eat it during the day also. I also mix Oil of Oregano with Apple Cider Vinegar and cold tea during the day just to get some Oil Of Oregano inside me as it is terribly strong and Apple Cider Vinegar is not the easiest thing to drink too. From looking at the blogs about giardia most people follow a sort of natural health protocol where as I just use what helps to stop the beast, so maybe I better get a protocol together.

Return To Vietnam

My diarrhea was controllable so I headed back to Vietnam to go back to teaching. I took my little bottle of Oil Of Oregano with me as well as a bottle of zinc tablets and Vitamin C 1000mg tablets. The rest I figured I could buy in Vietnam. The problem with buying medicine in Vietnam is the dosage is very low. Some pills the dosage was so low it was nearly useless. The Vitamin B multi were so low it was ridiculous so I brought them as single units like B12 and B6. Vitamin C was OK at 500mgs each so that is what I used. A lot of what I was eating before I just could not get in Vietnam. They had there own food and I could get Apple Cider Vinegar and coconut oil from the supermarket. My body was controllable so I didn't have too many problems. I could survive with the beast and live quite normally. In Vietnam they make really good bread so I was back on the bread very soon after I got there. Also I like pickled food and there is a lot of pickled food in the supermarket including a lot of

Asia pickles like pickled bamboo shoots which are very good. Vietnam is an eating-out society so a lot of people eat, but they love MSG and I mean they love it. The MSG aisle in the supermarket is the possibly the longest aisle in the supermarket, and for that reason I didn't like eating out too much, but I had to. I could get good garlic from the street markets and I ate Vitamin C with garlic very regularly like most nights. I had to eat Vit C as I couldn't get cucumin and spices were a terrible price as they were all imported.

I settled in very well, running around the lake in the morning and doing exercises in the park. The pollution was pretty bad and I was worried as I ran out of puff running in the mornings and I blamed it on the pollution. But it was actually food related and after I started eating avocados I could run a lot further. Everything was going OK and then one day for no apparent reason my planters fasciitis damaged foot just swelled up to about double the size. I was worried but as it was my planters fasciitis foot and I might have damaged it while running I didn't think it was serious, and it just meant there was a lot of inflammation in my body. So I overdosed on Vit C and popped my foot up high on pillows and waited, and as it didn't get any bigger I just left it and over-night it went down so it was only swollen up for about 24 hours. That was a worry but it was not serious, I just had to lay off the running for a couple of days, I could still do exercises as there was very little strain on my feet. My running schedule is cardio running one morning about 10kms, and HIIT the next morning for about 20 minutes and standard exercises, push-ups, squats, lunges, sit-ups and leg raises and the plank. I could do some of the exercises without putting too much strain on my foot.

My main line of defence against the beast was crushed and chopped garlic with Vitamin C last thing at night. I would crush and chop the garlic, about 4 to 5 big cloves, and leave sit for about 20 minutes then I would just swallow it as fast as possible to try and keep the smell down. Then I would take around 1000 to 1500 mgs of Vit C and go to bed, and leave that sit in my stomach all night. And it helped control the beast. Also as I was in the tropics I could eat as much papaya and papaya seeds as I wanted and the seeds help to kill the beast.

In Vietnam I had controllable diarrhea the whole time I was there. I could live with it within reason, but I just got tired of it.

Now before I left to go to Vietnam I noticed a brown mole on the side of my forehead start to get larger and after I got to Vietnam it had turned into a hard lump with a hole in the middle. I went to my doctor and he wanted to do a biopsy and cut it out. Anyway Vietnam will never be a medical tourist destination as it is incredibly expensive to see a doctor, so I didn't push the matter. Instead I went back to China and saw my Chinese Medicine Doctor. I used to work in China so I knew some doctors and they are a lot cheaper than in Vietnam. He gave me an iodine mix and told me to rub it hard into the lump. The key was rubbing the iodine mix hard into the lump and I didn't rub hard enough, so nothing happened. It just got a little bigger, so after about 6 weeks I was a bit worried so I started rubbing the q-tip a lot harder into the hard lump. And three months after I noticed the lump it started to get smaller then it went away, but it has since come back a few times and I have had to rub the iodine mix all over again but it didn't last very long and it faded away. I had basal skin cancer which is not very serious except it can get quite large. It is also called rodent bite cancer as the cancer has a hole in the middle like a rat bite.

I don't know if the skin cancer was caused by giardia or inflammation or the fact that my immune system was working overtime to keep the giardia under control or whatever. But it seems strange with the timing so when you have giardia just be careful as your body is under attack all the time and you never know what other aliments you might end up with.

Now Vietnam will never become a medical tourist destination as I said before, mainly because Thailand is next door and is already an established medical tourist destination. And it you are in Vietnam and you need an operation you just go to Thailand. But Vietnam is already a Dental tourist destination, that is why I first came here. I had a dental tooth implant from start to finish under $1000 US – that was from getting the tooth pulled out to the finished implant. The biggest problem was finding a dentist as there are dentists everywhere. I asked on facebook and somebody recommended this dentist and I went there and I'm glad I did. The dentists all spoke English and they are excellent. I had a problem with one of my teeth and my dentist in China didn't want to touch it and he had a Phd in Dentistry, and he was good. Also my dentist in my home town didn't want anything to do with it. And the Dentist in

Vietnam actually admitted it was not the usual procedure but he had done it before and said he would take my tooth out. And he did. Now every time I go to Vietnam I get my teeth checked.

Anyway depression sometimes invades as when you have the beast your life is controlled by the beast. So in one of my depressed states I wondered into the drug store and brought a packet of Tinidazole and took the standard 4 pills of 500mgs each and nothing happened, I was still the same. So a week later I took another 4 pills and nothing miraculous happened. Vietnam has some really good probiotics so I loaded up on those and regularly like everyday had my little sachet of probiotics mixed with water to try and get my stomach back to normal. I never seemed to be able to get my stomach back to what it was before Guardia, so maybe my doctor was right when he said I had IBS (Irritable Bowel Syndrome) I thought he was just trying to find something wrong with me because there was no giardia in my stool sample.

Just A Few Of My Thoughts On The Beast

I'm an English As A Second Language Teacher so I have spent a lot of time in developing countries and I have had my fair share of problems with different bugs. The worst case was Amoebic Dysentery in the Sahara and Flagyl saved my life. There I lost so much weight I was digging holes in my belt just to keep my pants up. Back then Flagyl was a carcinogenic and you couldn't drink alcohol when you were taking the medicine as it didn't mix too good. There seems to be a mixed response to Flagyl and a number of people have problems with it. When I used it the doctor stressed not to drink alcohol and now I don't know if the doctors still recommend no alcohol. It worked for me.

Giardia helped me lose faith in my doctor so now I try other doctors as well as natural health practitioners and I think that is a good idea. If your doctor is not looking after you go somewhere else. When I had a doctor look at my skin cancer he wanted to cut it out there and then without a biopsy so I went to another doctor.

Now with the internet I do my own research and learn as much as I can about what is wrong with me. But you have to be careful using the internet as you do not know if the information is correct or not, so check everything.

What I Used To Beat The Beast

17 ounces (500 grams) of Diatomaceous Earth Food Grade:
I used nearly all of this but it didn't stop the beast. It did stop my stomach from rumbling and I don't know if it killed stomach worms as I don't know if I had them.

35 ounces (1 kilogram) of Bentonite Clay Food Grade:
This was an asset and definitely helped kill the beast. I used about half the packet. You have to be careful with this product as it can block your intestines up. Leave it soaking over night, I used one tablespoon in a cup of water. Also near the end I would add a tablespoon of Psyllium Husk. Drink it before the Psyllium Husk swells up, and keep drinking fluids during the day. Also do not take any supplements or medication as the Bentonite Clay would soak them up and take them out of your body.

Heaps of Psyllium Husks preferably organic

Psyllium Husk is very healthy as it is nearly all fiber, that is if you just buy Psyllium Husk and not the mix I started with which was over half sugar. Be careful as it swells up and could block you up. Try it our first put a tablespoon in a glass then full with water then leave for about half an hour and you will find the Psyllium Husk would have soaked up all the water. So don't block yourself up. I used to leave it before eating to swell up and that way it would not swell up inside you, but I think it is better if you eat it and let it swell up inside you. This way you are soaking up the fluid in your stomach and hopefully that could help the diarrhea.

Cayenne Pepper

Excellent stuff you need this to kill the beast, but it is very hot so start small and increase the dose. In the end I was putting it on my dinner and mixing it with honey and coconut oil. I was probably eating around a small teaspoon a day. Just remember it is still hot when it comes out so don't go overboard.

Manuka Honey

This stuff is expensive but you need it. I read on the internet that there is a lot of under rated Manuka Honey out there so I stopped buying the most expensive and it was just as good. Any honey should do as it just gives the beast something to eat while it is also eating the Cayenne Pepper.

Coconut Oil Eating Oil

Not Cooking Oil preferable organic virgin
This is a must, you can mix it with Cayenne Pepper or just eat a big teaspoon a day

Lots of organic Garlic 4 cloves a night

This is a must as it kept me alive. It controlled the beast. I would eat it at night so it stayed in my stomach all night working its magic. I took it at night so I didn't smell so bad doing the day.

Tumeric

I used this to stop inflammation as I most definitely had some in my body, probably in my stomach where the beast was working overtime. Also because my foot took so long to heal I needed something for inflammation. I'm still using it

Vitamin C and Zinc to boost my immune system

Change Your Lifestyle And Eating Habits

You have to change what you do to survive work and after a very short time you will know where every public toilet is and which are the cleanest. The main rule is if you don't eat you don't run off to the toilet all the time. And if you are like me, you are convinced that drinking tea will send you to the toilet, and since you don't know which end is going to come out first, you sit down just in case.

Anyway I somehow evolved into this routine, I would go to bed earlier and get up earlier, like in bed before 10 and up before 5. This way I could clean myself out before going to work. Also my eating habits changed to fit my anti-beast health food regime. Like in the mornings after eating the Coconut Oil and Honey with Cayenne Pepper it is recommended to not eat or drink anything for 4 hours. So you have to stop eating, and if you eat Coconut Oil first then three to four hours later you eat the honey then you have to wait some more time. In the end I ate very little during the day, I just drank lots of tea then after work I would eat as much as I could early and about one and a half hours before I went to bed I would start on the garlic. On the weekends it was the same, very little food and lots of tea.

I evolved into this routine as it kept me at work and I could get through the day with minimal disruption. And I made sure I always had a wad of toilet paper stuffed up my butt and you will too. I actually thought about adult diapers, but didn't go that far.

A Few Things You Should Do

After using the toilet always put the seat down before you flush. It has been said when you flush the toilet very small water droplet get sprayed around the room and you don't want that. People keep saying that the antibiotics don't work and the beast seems to come back, but a lot of that could be reinfection. So be careful. Also when washing your hands after use do wash properly and rub the soap all over your hands. Actually antibiotic soap is not recommended as it kills all bacteria on your hands and you will be washing your hands more often as you go to the toilet more often. And try and keep your hands away from your face, this should help with stopping the reinfection. For drying your hands paper towels are better or cleaner than using a cloth towel. If you use a cloth towel wash it in very hot water as that should kill the beast.

One Thing You Must Do

You must stop eating sugar and any foods that turn to sugar in your body like bread, corn and rice as well as a number of other different foods. The beast loves sugar and you will find this out as I did, and I came to the conclusion that I was just wasting the anti-beast food that I was eating like Garlic, Cayenne Pepper and Manuka Honey when I was eating sugar. And most of the times I had very bad diarrhea was when I was eating sugar. So toss the sweets and sugar drinks until you have killed the beast then if possible don't go back on them again. It wont take you long to see the connection between sugar and diarrhea.

The Aftermath

I actually think I've managed to kill the beast. My criteria for being giardia free is slightly different from what my doctor would say. I would say I had the beast for well over a year. Tried everything mentioned in my book and I still don't know when it died off. If the doctor can't find anything in your poo sample they say you have IBS of leaky gut or some other gut related problem. And I never believed them because the symptoms didn't go away. But looking back I think they were right as my body had taken a hammering from the beast, so it should take a while to get back to normal and that took nearly another year.

My criteria for being beast free is

(1) I can fart without fear and anybody who has had the beast knows what I mean.

(2) Consistency and colour is back to normal

(3) I am regular like I used to be, Now all three are lined up but it has taken over 2 years to get back to normal.

What actually turned the tide for me was crushed raw garlic 4 to 5 cloves of good garlic - crushed, diced and leave sit for about 20 minutes plus 1000mgs to 1500 mgs of Vitamin C taken together every night last thing at night so it is on an empty stomach all night. But I still eat papaya seeds, cucumin to stop inflammation and Physillum Husk for fiber but not regular like the garlic. Now I can honestly say I feel better than I have felt for a long time.

Don't Panic If You Get Constipation

After I got over diarrhea I ended up with constipation. I'm not surprised really as I had spent over two years trying to hold everything in. And now it was time to reverse the situation, so I had to retrain my stomach muscles to force things out. That was a problem as my muscles had no strength so I couldn't force things out. So I started eating prunes, dates and other fiber foods like Physillum Husk and my muscles slowly returned to normal.

Don't panic and overdose on anti diarrhea meds as some are just not safe. Loperamide, which is marketed and sold as Imodium, is actually an opioid so be careful, very careful with this med. I used to live of this stuff, every time I went on a plane or a bus I loaded up with this med and I didn't realize how dangerous it is.

How I Ended Up on Garlic And Vitamin C

When I was in Vietnam one vitamin that is easy to buy with a good dosage is Vitamin C whereas a lot of vitamins and supplements have a very limited dosage. Some supplements only have 10% active ingredient so to get the same dosage as we get back home you need to take 10 tablets. And since the tablets are the same size as back home I wonder what the filler is. You are eating a lot of junk just to get the same dose. Also the tariffs on imported medicine must run about 200% as imported supplements are way expensive. And garlic is everywhere so it was easy to join the two together and it worked. So that is what I recommend.

If You Like My Book

Please write a review on Amazon showing your appreciation

How to Write a Review on Amazon

Go to https://www.amazon.com/dp/1095299891

Scroll down to Customer Reviews

- Click on "Write a customer review" and do your thing. As long or as short as you like.

Amazon will then check it and after a while it will be live on Amazon.

Now you can give the book a grade, how many Gold Stars would you like to give the book.

Thank you

Peter LeGrove

Other Books By Peter LeGrove

Teach and Travel in China

This little book is all about going to China and getting a job teaching English. Even though it is Guangzhou specific it still covers little things that could happen in China. A good read if you are heading out into the world to travel.

How To Teach Young Learners ESL

This book is an accumulation of my seven years of classroom teaching, face to face with kids from kindergarten to the end of primary school. This is what worked for me, and it has been distilled from lots of stuff that didn't work. So you end up with the crème de la crème. Teaching kids is the way to go, if you are into teaching and traveling.

Reading Student Struggling Student

If you are not into leaving your child in front of the computer to learn to read, then this book is for you. This is a hands on approach to teaching your child to read, using a method that has been teaching children to read for over a hundred years. And it is still applicable in this internet age.

How To Add Qualifications To Your CV

Using FREE Courses

To add more color to your CV, and to help give you the edge in the job market. Fill up the spaces with certificates from free courses run by world renowned universities. There is a whole new world of free education out there in cyberspace, you just have to plug into and this little book shows you where it all is.

How To Make An Online CV

Using Free Software

With the internet taking over our lives it is only a matter of time before you apply for an online job using an Online CV. In this little book you will learn how to put together a professional Online CV using only FREE software freely available over the internet. Also what you learn can be adapted to online presentations as well.

Prepare Your Children For The Future NOW

The world with the internet is changing so fast now it is very difficult to keep up. So to keep your children ahead of the curve you need to start them early on the internet. This way when they are ready to head out into the New World of cyberspace they are already over half way there.

Live Cheap In An UnCheap World

For some reason the world we live in is getting more and more expensive, so now it is time to change. To make your money last longer, you either have to tighten your belt, make more money or do things differently. Now this little books shows you ways to do all three so you can end up with more money at the end of the week.

Prepare Now To Survive Mother Nature's Wrath Or Mankind's Madness

At present in the world, there is a group of people who think the world is heading for a major collapse. And on the other side, there has been an increase in what Mother Nature can do to the planet. This book is about common sense preparing for what could happen without going overboard.

Live And Teach In Vietnam

If you are looking for country where you can "Live Cheap In An UnCheap World" then Vietnam should be on your radar. This little book tells you about life as it is on the streets of Vietnam, and how to get a job, place to stay and what ever else you need.

Thank you and all the best on your journey to rid yourself of internal stomach parasites. There is hope but sometimes it can seem to be a long way off.

Peter LeGrove